EASY WAYS TO MANAGE DIABETES

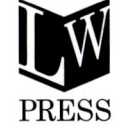

LW PRESS

Author: Jean Betschart, M.N., M.S.N., C.R.N.P., C.D.E.
Consulting Organization: The American Association of Diabetes Educators
Coordinating Consultant: Susan Thom, R.D., L.D., C.D.E.
Consultants: Kris Ernst, R.N., C.D.E.
Karmeen Kulkarni, M.S., R..D., C.D.E.
Marilyn Graff, B.S.N., R.N., C.D.E.
Richard Rubin, Ph.D., C.D.E.
Deborah Hinnen Hentzen, M.N., R.N., C.D.E.

This publication is for informational purposes and is not intended to provide medical advice. Neither Publications International, Ltd., nor the author, consultants, editors, or publisher take responsibility for any possible consequences from any treatment, procedure, exercise, dietary modification, action, or application of medication or preparation by any person reading or following the information in this publication. The publication of this book does not constitute the practice of medicine, and this publication does not attempt to replace your physician or other health care provider. Before undertaking any course of treatment, the author, consultants, editors, and publisher advise the reader to check with a physician or other health care provider.

The brand-name products mentioned in this publication are trademarks or service marks of their respective companies. The mention of any product in this publication does not constitute an endorsement by Publications International, Ltd., nor does it constitute an endorsement by any of these companies that their products should be used in the manner recommended by this publication.

Copyright © 2006 LW Press. All rights reserved. This book may not be reproduced or quoted in whole or in part by any means whatsoever without written permission from:

LW Press, a division of
Publications International, Ltd.
Louis Weber, CEO
7373 North Cicero Avenue
Lincolnwood, Illinois 60712

Permission is never granted for commercial purposes.

Manufactured in China.

8 7 6 5 4 3 2 1

ISBN: 1-4127-1311-0

CONTENTS

Introduction 5

1. Fit Diabetes into Your Life!............ 6
2. Assemble a Winning Team.............. 8
3. Take the Helm 10
4. Make It a Family Affair 11
5. Teach Your Friends 13
6. Gear Up!........................... 15
7. Put Two and Two Together 18
8. Stick to a Routine................... 20
9. Test Without Fail 23
10. Take Medicine Properly.............. 26
11. Write It Down 28
12. Exercise!........................... 29
13. Plan Your Diet...................... 30
14. Be a Label Reader................... 33
15. Lean Away from Fat 35
16. Fit in Fiber......................... 36

17. Know How Alcohol Fits In 37

18. Plan for Parties 38

19. Pamper Your Feet 40

20. See Your Eye Doctor. 42

21. Adjust for Sick Days 43

22. Don't Give Your Mouth the Brush-Off 45

23. Identify Yourself 47

24. Safeguard Your Sex Life 48

25. Maintain Tight Control for Pregnancy 50

26. Look Out for Lows 52

27. Watch for Ketones. 55

28. Store Your Insulin Properly 56

29. Be Prepared! 58

30. Look for Patterns 59

31. Advocate for Your Needs on the Job 62

32. Drive Safely 63

33. Carpe Diem: Seize the Day! 64

INTRODUCTION

Most of the time, we have a pretty good idea what we should do to maintain our health and well-being. The hard part is actually doing it. We're familiar with the drill: Brush and floss our teeth, exercise regularly, reduce fat and cholesterol, reduce stress, limit alcohol intake, see the doctor for checkups. But how many of us consistently perform these healthy habits? The answer is, very few! So it's no surprise that it is equally—if not more—difficult to manage diabetes consistently.

We know the tasks persons with diabetes must perform: take medication, test blood glucose levels, follow a prescribed meal plan, exercise regularly, and keep accurate and current records. Doing it all is tough! And it's especially hard if we think we may need to perform these tasks for the rest of our lives. So why keep up with them at all?

Research has proved that control of blood glucose levels can markedly decrease the risk of diabetes-related complications such as blindness and kidney disease in people with insulin-dependent diabetes. It can also slow their advance in people who already have signs of these conditions. Therefore, experts believe all people with diabetes should manage their blood glucose levels to protect their future health and well-being.

Since you're reading this book, you've decided to recruit the help you need to remove the obstacles and fit diabetes into your life. Remember, diabetes control doesn't happen overnight. It's a process—and you won't be perfect at it every day. But, as this book reminds you, you won't be alone either. Others have been successful—you can be, too.

1

FIT DIABETES INTO YOUR LIFE!

Let's be honest. It's not easy to fit diabetes into your life without making it the center of your existence. The people who accomplish this seem to perform their diabetes tasks quietly, not making a big deal about them. They test their blood glucose routinely, adjusting their meals, activity, or diabetes medication according to their schedule. They have learned to work diabetes into their lifestyle. To them, diabetes care comes as naturally as brushing their teeth each morning. If you're having trouble getting on track with diabetes management, try these tips:

• Stock the proper tools. Keep plenty of diabetes supplies, such as lancets, testing strips for blood and urine, diabetes medication, syringes, and glucose tablets or juice, on hand. Make sure you have replacement batteries for your glucose meter and an extra pen for recording your blood glucose results. A travel or cosmetics case can keep supplies together, organized, and portable. Consider having two meters, one at home and one at work for easy access.

• Purchase appropriate foods to make diabetes care easy for you. If you must buy desserts and other temptations for your family, store them out of sight. Temptation that stares you in the face is hard to resist.

• If you find yourself in a slump with your care, enlist the support of family and friends to remind you to keep up with your testing and medication. Bear in mind your testing does not become their responsibility; it is yours.

• Devise ways to remind yourself. Leave your meter in an obvious location so you remember to test. Leave yourself notes in conspicuous places. Synchronize the testing and/or medication to coincide with other activities in your daily routine; for example, when the coffee is brewing in the morning, test your blood glucose.

• Establish a routine. It sounds so obvious, but if you establish a routine for your care, diabetes management becomes an automatic response, even when you feel stressed or pressured by other events in your life.

• Don't let diabetes care keep you from doing something you really want to do. With frequent testing and a good understanding of your diabetes care, you can participate in most activities you enjoy.

2

ASSEMBLE A WINNING TEAM

One of the most important elements of a successful diabetes care program is a health care provider. Whether you work with one professional or a team of professionals, you should feel your health care provider is willing to listen to your concerns and take the time to make sure you understand how best to manage diabetes.

Your doctor may be an endocrinologist, a doctor who specializes in dealing with hormonal problems. (Insulin is a hormone.) A child or adolescent with diabetes may be cared for by a pediatric endocrinologist who has special knowledge about diabetes in children. If an endocrinologist is not available in your area, choose a doctor who has experience in diabetes care. Ultimately, a physician's most important qualification is that you feel comfortable with him or her.

Ideally, a multidisciplinary team is available to you. The team may include a doctor, nurse educator, registered dietitian, social worker, psychologist or psychiatrist, and exercise physiologist. But all of these specialists may not be available in the area in which you live or the health care setting you use. You and your doctor may need to put together your own team:

• Ask your doctor to refer you to a diabetes educator or dietitian. The American Association of Diabetes Educators can also provide you with names; phone them at 1-800-338-3633 or visit their Web site at www.aadnet.org and click on Diabetes Education in the left menu, then select "Find a Diabetes Educator."

• Look for professionals with the credential C.D.E, which stands for Certified Diabetes Educator. This abbreviation assures you that this licensed provider has met certain educational requirements and has passed an examination that verifies knowledge and expertise in diabetes.

Finding a health care professional who is sensitive to your needs and able to provide the support you need is critical to your diabetes care. Communication is vital: Are you comfortable talking with this person? Is he or she readily available and willing to take time to answer questions or help with medication adjustments? You may need to talk with a few health care professionals before you find one who is right for you.

3

TAKE THE HELM

With health care systems changing, it's up to you to steer the direction of your care. If you're unsure how to be an advocate for yourself, here are a few suggestions:

• Don't settle for someone who will not work with you to keep diabetes under optimal control. If a health care provider is too busy to spend time with you or seems unaware of how best to help you, find someone else. Even if you've been seeing one physician for a long time, do not feel compelled to stick with him or her. A physician who is unable to help you because of patient load or lack of experience with diabetes is not the best physician for you, no matter how long you've known him or her.

• Ask your physician to refer you to a diabetes educator, registered dietitian, and/or psychologist if you have difficulty in areas where these professionals can help. And don't feel put out or dismissed if your physician refers you to one of these professionals without your asking. A physician who recognizes that others can help where he or she cannot is putting your needs first.

• Tell your health care provider what part of your management program you can do easily and where you have difficulty. Together you can come up with ideas to smooth over the rocky areas and reinforce the strong areas.

• Stay abreast of new research and developments in diabetes care. Ask your health care provider if new products might benefit you.

• Demand frequent communication with your health care provider so he or she can carefully monitor your blood glucose levels.

MAKE IT A FAMILY AFFAIR

Diabetes is called a family disease because it affects every family member. Food selection and preparation as well as the timing of meals are important aspects of family life. The need for medication and avoidance of hypoglycemia (low blood glucose) can take away some spontaneity from meals. And dining out presents a whole new challenge.

Your diabetes management affects your family in other ways, too. They undoubtedly have feelings about your health, ranging from concern and sympathy to guilt and resentment. They may also worry about their own susceptibility to diabetes. Perhaps your treatment affects your family financially. Perhaps you require your family's help to pick up (or even administer) your medication or drive you to appointments with your doctor or diabetes educator. Recognize that the more your family members know about diabetes control, the more you all benefit. To get your family involved:

• Ask family members to attend diabetes education classes with you. Their direct participation will involve them more effectively than a simple explanation of what was taught, and they will have the opportunity to ask questions of the instructor. Discuss what each of you learned, and ask your educator to clarify any discrepancies.

• Provide your family with reading materials. Encourage them to join the American Diabetes Association.

• Practice skills at home with your family: Perform finger sticks for blood glucose, inject saline into an orange or doll, and review the treatment for hypoglycemia so family members can understand what you go through and also carry out these acts in case of emergency.

• Make sure family members know your meal and medication schedule. Tell them how you plan to handle any schedule changes so they're prepared in the event of complications.

• Encourage any family member who is having trouble coping with your having diabetes to seek counseling to discuss his or her feelings.

Teach Your Family:

- What diabetes is
- The types of diabetes
- How diabetes is treated
- Your individualized treatment plan
- The importance of meal planning, preparation, and timing
- About your medications (how to inject insulin, if appropriate)
- The signs of hypoglycemia
- The treatment for hypoglycemia and where you keep supplies
- Your plan of record keeping
- How to help with sick days
- Emergency phone numbers

5

TEACH YOUR FRIENDS

Some people are reluctant to tell others about their diabetes care needs. But friends who care can help you stay on top of your program. Friends will take their attitude about diabetes from you. If you see it as a stigma, they may be reluctant to help you. On the other hand, if they see you taking charge of your condition and talking about it openly and honestly, they will feel more confident about helping you remain in control.

Friends won't know how they can support you unless you tell them. Here are ways to help your friends understand the role of diabetes in your life:

• Let others know how they can help you: "It really helps me when I see you order healthy foods off the menu first...." Let them know how you feel about them eating sweet foods and desserts in front of you. Some people find it difficult not to eat what everyone else has; others don't mind at all when their friends have sweet foods. Clear the air with your friends, and cast off everyone's uncertainty about what to do.

• Encourage your friends to jump on the bandwagon. Everyone can—and should—eat a low-fat, well-balanced diet, exercise, and control their weight. Explain that just because you have diabetes, you needn't eat foods that are "different" than everyone else. The healthful behaviors you adopt to control diabetes and your weight are elements of a healthy lifestyle everyone can participate in.

• Describe the signs and symptoms of hypoglycemia (low blood glucose) and how to treat it. Show friends where you keep treatment supplies, such as glucose tablets, juice, candy, or a Glucagon emergency kit, and explain how much of each you should receive in the event you do not recognize the signs yourself.

• Show friends where you carry emergency phone numbers. Keep a list posted near your phone so visitors can find the numbers easily.

• Engage your friends in diabetes-related activities through the American Diabetes Association or Juvenile Diabetes Association International. Ask friends to participate in a fund-raiser walk with you.

Tell Your Friends:

- The signs and symptoms of hypoglycemia
- How you treat hypoglycemia
- Where you keep supplies
- Emergency phone numbers
- How you plan to manage meals, diabetes medication, and so forth around special events
- The importance of eating on time
- Other ways you would like them to participate in your diabetes management

6

GEAR UP!

A variety of supplies are available to help you care for diabetes. Most likely, you will choose your equipment based on the recommendations of your physician or educator, the cost, and your personal preferences. If your drugstore does not carry the supplies you need or want, ask the pharmacist to order them. You can also order equipment and supplies by mail. Here's a look at some of the supplies you need.

Meters to Measure Blood Glucose Levels

Ask your diabetes educator to recommend a meter that is appropriate for your needs. Most meters last three to four years. Prices will vary, as will their individual features. Consider buying two meters if you are on the go a lot—one for home and one for your purse, briefcase, backpack, or desk. Before you purchase a meter, consider the following:

• Do you need a meter with a memory? Some meters store the date, time, and result of previous blood glucose tests; some also give your average blood glucose level. Some meters have no memory.

• How quickly do you need results? Depending on the meter, it can take from 6 seconds to 2 minutes to obtain results.

• How do you maintain the meter? Is cleaning necessary? How difficult is it to clean?

• How many steps does testing require; that is, do you need to do timing, wiping, or other additional steps that make testing complicated?

• Will the meter tell you when something is wrong—not enough blood, a dirty window, poor timing? Can it still yield accurate results despite some minor imperfections in your testing technique?

• Is it easy to calibrate the meter to the type of testing strips you have?

• What kind of batteries (if any) does it have? How often do they need to be replaced? (Generally, batteries should be good for at least 1,000 tests.)

• How large is the meter? Can you carry it in a pocket or purse?

• Does the manufacturer provide technical support in case you have a problem with the meter? Does the manufacturer have a toll-free number for customer service?

• What is the cost of the strips the meter uses? (Your doctor or educator may recommend generic strips.)

Lancets to Obtain Blood for Testing

Lancets vary according to the size of the point and the depth of penetration. Some are designed for children or people with especially sensitive fingers.

• Ask your diabetes educator to give you a variety of lancets to sample. All meters come with finger-prick devices, and you can use most lancets with most devices.

• If you use a lancing device, check to see if its end-cap (the end that covers the lancet) has holes of different diameters to let the lancet through. This features allows you to adjust the end-cap for calloused fingers so you can obtain a deeper puncture and thus a better blood sample.

Remember: Never share your finger-pricking device without first cleaning the end-cap with a bleach solution. End-caps can transmit blood-borne viruses such as hepatitis or human immunodeficiency virus (HIV), the virus that causes AIDS. And never share lancets.

Syringes for Injecting Insulin

The size of the syringe you use depends on your maximum dose of insulin. Insulin is measured in units. Insulin syringes come in 30-, 50-, and 100-unit sizes. The needles for each are the same size; the numbers correspond to the size of the barrel of the syringe. When purchasing syringes, allow about 15 percent extra space in the event you need to increase your dose of insulin. If your usual dose is 50 units, buy 100-unit syringes so you're prepared if your doctor increases your dose to, say, 53 units.

Many people safely reuse their insulin syringes. After an injection, they simply recap the syringe and store it with their insulin. Do not do this if there is any chance someone else might be stuck with the needle. However, if you require two or three injections a day, you can use one syringe for the day and then discard it.

Medical Waste

Be sure to follow this advice for handling used equipment:

- Dispose of your syringes and lancets in a tightly capped, well-labeled container.
- Call your township, city, or borough for information regarding disposal of medical waste in your area.

7
PUT TWO AND TWO TOGETHER

Until it becomes second nature, you must think about how medication, food, exercise, stress, illness, and other variables work together to affect your blood glucose level. Understanding the balance can be complex, but it is vital to diabetes management. And even once you understand and incorporate the balance, you may be frustrated to find your glucose levels are still not where you want them to be.

Here are some factors that may cause blood glucose levels to rise and fall:

Makes Glucose Levels Go Up	Makes Glucose Levels Go Down
Food	Missed, delayed, or inadequate meal
Stress	Exercise
Not enough medication	Diabetes medication

Every element in one column corresponds with an element in the other. For example, exercise lowers blood glucose levels, so one way to balance the level is to eat more.

The type of insulin you take also plays a significant role. Insulin has a peak action time—the time it has its strongest effect on your blood glucose levels. Each kind of insulin works differently. To keep track of all the factors that contribute to diabetes control:

• Test your blood glucose before and after you eat or exercise more than usual, and record any impact.

• Track how your blood glucose level responds to different foods. For example, see how the level increases after you eat similar amounts of potatoes, pasta, or corn. Do the same with similar foods: Compare sugar-sweetened cereals to unsweetened cereals.

• Highlight high or low blood glucose levels on your record sheets in different colors. See if high or low blood glucose values correspond to the peak action times of insulin(s).

• Share the information from frequent testing with your health professional so together you can fine-tune your management.

8

STICK TO A ROUTINE

One of the most helpful strategies to control blood glucose levels is sticking to a schedule. Granted, it isn't always easy to stick to a routine in our busy lives, but there are many reasons to try. Maintaining a consistent schedule of eating, exercise, and use of medication helps to identify patterns of highs and lows in your blood glucose records so you can adjust your program for better control.

If you have type II diabetes, and diet and exercise are your means of diabetes control, it is less important for you to follow a schedule rigidly. However, if you use an insulin pump or a multiple daily injection plan (three or more injections a day), you may already have more flexibility in your schedule.

Try these techniques for creating a feasible schedule:

• Write down your normal daily routine. With your diabetes educator's help, identify changes that could help you obtain better control. For example, if you notice your blood glucose runs too low on days you play tennis, you may need to reduce your medication or eat more on those days.

• Establish a daily exercise time, whether morning, afternoon, or evening. Many people find they have the most energy and get the most out of exercise when they exercise early in the morning. In addition, blood glucose does not fall quite as easily in response to morning exercise. If you have type I diabetes, you may need to exercise after breakfast to ensure that your blood glucose level doesn't drop too low.

• If you know your schedule will change for a week or even a day and you're unsure how to fit diabetes management in, consult your educator or doctor. For example, your child's soccer game or that pro basketball game you finally got tickets for may overlap with the supper hour; you're attending an afternoon wedding and the meal will be served at 3 P.M.; or your family is gathering for Mother's Day brunch at 10 A.M. With a little strategizing, these schedule shifts can fit in smoothly.

• Try to stay within 1 to 1½ hours of your regular schedule.

• Try to wake about the same time every day—even on weekends. If you get up at 6:30 during the week and 10:30 on weekends, you may wake on those late mornings with a blood glucose level that is too high or too low. Also, because you're starting your day later than usual, you're likely to throw off all your meal times or end up compressing your meals into a shorter overall period. Diabetes control requires a balance. When you make a change in one area, such as in your schedule or in amounts of food or exercise, you may need to adjust one of the other elements. What you adjust is up to you; there are no rules. If sleeping late causes a pattern of high blood glucose at lunch, you could: 1) eat less at breakfast; 2) eat lunch later; 3) increase Regular insulin in the morning; 4) exercise in the morning. Or you may need to select a combination of these approaches. Be sure to cover the peak times of your medications with a snack. And don't give yourself the next shot until the medication you took previously has peaked.

• If you want to change your regular schedule for some reason, such as a vacation, alter your schedule gradually, testing your blood glucose level frequently. Try moving your morning diabetes medication and breakfast a half hour later each day until you get on your new schedule. Again, look for a pattern of high or low blood glucose over three or four days. If a pattern develops, you may need to adjust food, medication, exercise, or your schedule.

• Try to keep food quantities and types of foods consistent. The greater the consistency, the better you can predict how your blood glucose will respond.

• Develop a routine for insulin injections. For example, take all injections in your abdomen. Or take morning injections in your arms, evening injections in your legs. This technique helps cut down on variability of insulin absorption that can occur when you use different sites.

TEST WITHOUT FAIL

Testing your blood glucose levels is your most valuable tool for determining how successful you are at diabetes control. And thanks to current technology, testing is easy. True, most people will never enjoy poking their finger for a drop of blood, but the new lancets make this step more comfortable. And the newest meters, which are small, portable, convenient, and fast, can make the rest of the testing process absolutely painless.

Tips for Performing the Finger Stick

Still make a face every time you do a finger stick? Believe it or not, you will get used to it. Rotate fingers. Experiment with sites. And follow these tips for smooth and uniform finger sticks:

• Wash your hands. Clean fingers reduce the risk of infection, but cleanliness also ensures accuracy of test results. Soap and water is fine for cleansing. Alcohol in single-use packets is a good choice when soap and water are not handy but not a good choice for everyday use. Alcohol can dry the skin and, if not wiped away, can cause a false-high reading when it mixes with blood. Dry your hands thoroughly.

• Warm your hands to increase blood supply to the area. Hang them down, shake them, or wash them in warm water. Milk the finger from the base to the tip to increase blood flow to the fingertip.

• Anchor your finger on a tabletop. You'll be less likely to get a stick that is too shallow.

• Use the sides of your fingers and thumbs. These areas are less sensitive but rich in capillary blood.

Tips for Meter Use

Once you've selected a meter suitable for your needs, follow this advice:

• Keep lancets, alcohol (if necessary for out-of-the-way testing locations), testing strips, and your record sheet together.

• Check your meter's accuracy frequently. Change the code, calibration chip, or strip when appropriate. (You need to adjust your meter to match each bottle or box of strips you use.) The meter comes with instructions for performing this simple procedure.

When to Test Blood Glucose

When you test depends on your doctor's recommendations. If you do not take diabetes medication, you may not need to test as often as someone who does. At least two days per week, you should test in the morning before breakfast and perhaps just before or two hours after each meal. If you take diabetes medication, especially if you use an intensive insulin routine involving multiple daily injections or an insulin pump, you need to test much more frequently—usually before each meal and at bedtime. Follow these general guidelines for testing:

• Test anytime you do not feel right. Low blood glucose may be the cause of a headache, hunger, unusual fatigue, weakness, shakiness, or inability to concentrate. These are also symptoms of anxiety and normal hunger, however, so it's important to test.

• Test before and after eating foods you suspect cause your glucose level to run high or low. Then the next time you eat that food, you can adjust your insulin or the amount you eat.

- Once a week, test your glucose during the night—say, between 2 and 4 A.M.
- Test frequently when you are sick. If you are vomiting or are very ill, test at least every two hours and perform a urine ketone test at least every 24 hours.
- Test before driving a vehicle. Test every two hours during car trips.
- Test if you're unsure whether to eat. If you're dining out and dinner might be late, a test can help you decide if you should have a snack.
- Test during the peak action times of your insulin. For example, Regular insulin peaks two to four hours after injection. Therefore, if you take Regular insulin at 7 A.M., you might test your blood around 9:30 or 10 A.M.
- Test before and after you exercise. Glucose levels can continue to fall for up to 24 hours after strenuous exercise, even after an insulin injection.

10

TAKE MEDICINE PROPERLY

Whether you take insulin injections or an oral agent (pill) to lower your blood glucose, it is critical that you take the right dose at the right time. Make sure you know the type and dose of your medication, when it starts to lower blood glucose, when it works hardest (peaks), and how long it is effective.

If you take an oral agent:

• Ask your diabetes educator or doctor what to do if you miss a dose. If you completely miss a dose, do not double up on your next dose.

• Know if you should take your medication on an empty stomach or with food.

• Learn to recognize the signs of hypoglycemia (low blood glucose).

• Report any side effects, such as stomach problems or rashes, to your doctor.

If you take insulin, your diabetes educator will show you the proper technique for giving yourself an insulin injection. Each time you give yourself a shot, keep the following in mind:

• Roll NPH, Lente, or Ultralente insulin to mix it before drawing it up into the syringe.

• Always draw air into the syringe in the amount of your dose, and inject this air into the insulin bottle. Replacing the insulin you remove with air prevents the airtight bottle from developing a vacuum. If you don't perform this step, it will become more difficult to remove the insulin each time.

Easy Ways to Manage Diabetes

- If you mix insulins, always do it in the same order so you do not confuse your doses. For example, draw up Regular into the syringe first, then NPH.
- Check for air bubbles. If injected into your skin, an air bubble will not hurt you, but its presence probably means you're not getting the correct dose of insulin. If you see a bubble, push the insulin back into the bottle and draw it up again.
- Make sure you've measured accurately. If necessary, ask a family member or friend to double-check your dose. If you have trouble seeing the lines on the syringe, try holding it in front of something white. If this technique doesn't help, magnifiers that clamp around the syringe are available at most pharmacies.
- Pinch the skin where you wish to inject the insulin. Inject insulin straight in at a 90-degree angle.
- If you have trouble with insulin leaking at injection sites, pull the skin to one side before inserting the needle and count to 10 before pulling the needle out. Make sure to release the pinched skin before pulling the needle out. The pressure of the pinch can force insulin out the hole.
- If occasionally you find it hard to push the insulin in, pull the needle back a bit and try again. If it still does not plunge, start again with a new syringe.
- If you have frequent bruising or unusual pain at your injection sites, let your diabetes educator or doctor watch your injection technique.

11

WRITE IT DOWN

Keeping records of every test, every result, every dose, every symptom, and every sign is one of the best ways for you and your doctor to assess the success of diabetes control. Excellent record keeping allows you to identify patterns of high and low blood glucose levels, the effects of certain foods, and your body's response to exercise.

Here are some guidelines that will help make record keeping easier:

• Keep your record and a pen or pencil near your meter or, if possible, inside the carrying case so you are more likely to fill it in immediately. Don't rely on memory (yours or the meter's) to catch up on your record keeping.

• If you have an active day, either at work or play, make a note of this. When you look back in your record, these notes can help explain why numbers were a bit lower than usual that day.

• If you are sick, if you eat more or less than you usually do, or if your schedule was off on any given day, write this down.

• If you experience low blood glucose and treat for it, write this down.

• Write down any blood glucose results you obtain in between your usual test times, any additional insulin doses, and use of any other medication—prescription or over the counter—such as antibiotics or cold remedies.

• Study your records periodically. Are the numbers where you want them to be? Do you see any patterns?

• Always take your records with you to doctor appointments.

EXERCISE!

There's no doubt exercise greatly benefits people with diabetes. Regular exercise lowers blood glucose and cholesterol levels; reduces your risk of high blood pressure, heart attack, and stroke; and improves bone. If you are overweight or older than 40 years of age, however, check with your doctor before you begin an exercise program.

• Schedule a regular time to exercise.

• Warm up before and cool down after any exercise session. Perform stretches as well as light aerobic exercises to get the blood moving into your muscles.

• Wear comfortable gear appropriate for the temperature and activity. Wear thick or even double socks if you are prone to blisters.

• Test blood glucose levels before and after exercise. If you usually exercise for longer than 30 minutes, and your blood glucose is usually in your target range, plan to eat more before, during, and after exercise. If you take insulin, you can also consider adjusting your dose before exercise.

• Always have a simple sugar handy in case you experience low blood glucose. Eat it if you feel unusually uncoordinated, sweaty, or light-headed. When you exercise strenuously or for a long period, take a break for some juice or a snack to keep your blood glucose levels up. In general, eat 15 grams of carbohydrate for each hour of moderate activity.

• Drink plenty of water before, during, and after exercising.

• Ask your doctor or diabetes educator about exercise precautions when your insulin is peaking, when you have ketones in your urine, or when you exercise more than two hours after eating.

13

PLAN YOUR DIET

Thoughtful meal planning has always been the cornerstone of diabetes treatment. If you have type II diabetes, nutrition planning may be your only course of treatment. If you require a pill or insulin, you must balance your medication and exercise therapy with meal planning.

But if you thought that having diabetes meant you could never again enjoy a dish of ice cream, you may be in for a very pleasant surprise. In May 1994, the American Diabetes Association and the American Dietetic Association drafted new nutrition guidelines for the management of diabetes. The new guidelines prescribe a diet based on an individual's metabolism, lifestyle, and nutritional needs instead of the traditional calorie-based plan. The goals of the new guidelines are to help people with diabetes achieve a reasonable weight and normal blood glucose levels, lipid levels (particularly cholesterol and triglycerides), and blood pressure.

The new nutrition guidelines may also make your life a little sweeter. They emphasize total carbohydrate intake—whether the carbohydrate source is sugar or starch, cake or mashed potatoes. Research has demonstrated that all carbohydrates end up as glucose; it's just a matter of time. So nutrition experts now consider all carbohydrates as one food category. You may consume some sugary foods in place of some starchy foods as long as you don't exceed your recommended total intake of carbohydrate for the day or meal.

You should work with a registered dietitian to create a meal plan tailored to your current and desirable body

Easy Ways to Manage Diabetes

weight, eating and exercise patterns, blood glucose and hemoglobin A1c records, and any medication you take.

There are three main eating plans recommended to help people with diabetes. They are:

• The exchange system. This sytem allows you to eat a wide variety of foods while keeping blood glucose levels stable. You work with a registered dietitian to design a diet based on a series of exchanges. Each food is assigned to one of six different groups. Each food in the group turns into an approximately equal amount of glucose. You're permitted a certain number of food exchanges from various categories for each meal. The dietitian helps you determine the number of exchanges you should eat each day.

• Carbohydrate counting. In this system, you're permitted a certain amount of carbohydrates per day and per meal. You'll work with a registered dietitian to determine how many carbohydrate grams you should eat at each meal and snack to keep blood glucose close to normal. Many people find carb counting easier than the exchange system. Whenever possible, choose high-fiber, whole-grain products, beans, and fresh fruits and vegetables.

• The diabetic food pyramid. This pyramid offers daily recommendations for the number of servings you should have per food group. It allows small amounts of fats, sweets, and alcohol. Talk with a registered dietitian for specific recommendations that are best for you if the pyramid approach appeals to you.

Here are some tips for a successful meal plan:

• Determine your most important goal in managing diabetes and planning your diet. Do you want to lose weight? Make more nutritious food choices? Tell your

Easy Ways to Manage Diabetes

registered dietitian your goals and in what areas you need the most help.

• Check your progress. Monitor blood glucose, hemoglobin A_{1C} results, lipid levels, and any weight loss.

• Keep good records. Identify areas where you're doing well and where you're having difficulty.

• Maintain a regular schedule. Consistency in timing and amount of food is important for people who require insulin. You must also learn to balance food with the actions of insulin on days when your schedule changes or when you are more or less active than usual.

• Space meals and snacks throughout the day, instead of eating only three meals.

• Lose weight if you need to. Extra body fat makes it harder for the body to produce insulin to match your intake of food. As a result, you require more insulin to balance glucose levels. Weight loss allows the insulin to work more effectively. Many people have decreased their insulin dose after weight loss.

BE A LABEL READER

If you haven't noticed, food package labels are now worthwhile reading. A gift to consumers from our federal friends, the Nutrition Labeling and Education Act of 1990 requires manufacturers to put specific nutrition information on food labels. The labels make it easy to select foods that fit into your meal plan. The labels list, for one serving, the nutrients most relevant to your health: total and saturated fats, cholesterol, sodium, carbohydrates, dietary fiber, sugars, proteins, and vitamins and minerals. Serving sizes are now standardized to help you make better-informed choices. The % Daily Value column shows how this food fits into a daily diet of 2,000 calories.

The nutrition label is not the only label you should understand. What about other claims on labels? Claims on product labels must meet legal standards set by the government. Here's a dictionary of claims:

If the label says:	The product contains, per serving:
Sugar free	less than ½ gram of sugar
Nonfat or Fat free	½ gram of fat or less
Low fat	3 grams of fat or less
Reduced fat	25% less saturated fat than similar foods
Lean	less than 10 grams of fat, 4 grams of saturated fat, and 95 milligrams of cholesterol

Extra lean	less than 5 grams of fat, 2 grams of saturated fat, and 95 milligrams of cholesterol
Calorie free	less than 5 calories
Low calorie	40 calories or less
Reduced calorie	At least 25% fewer calories than similar foods
Light or Lite	⅓ fewer calories or 50% less fat
Low cholesterol	20 milligrams or less cholesterol and 2 grams or less saturated fat
Cholesterol free	Less than 2 milligrams cholesterol and 2 grams or less saturated fat
High fiber	5 grams of fiber or more

Talk to your dietitian to learn more about fitting different foods into your meal plan. Save the labels from foods you have questions about so your dietitian can help you figure out how to plug them into your meal plan.

A caution to those who use the American Diabetes Association Exchange List: The standard serving sizes listed on the product label may differ from the size listed on the exchange list. For example, a standard serving size of fruit juice is 8 ounces, but the exchange lists a fruit juice serving size as 4 ounces.

LEAN AWAY FROM FAT

People with diabetes are three times more likely to develop heart disease. One factor contributing to that increased risk is the high blood cholesterol common among people with type 2 diabetes. Research suggests you should choose a diet with less than 30 percent of calories coming from fat—and very little of that from saturated and trans fats.

How do you start? First, pay attention to the type of fat you eat. Read labels; they indicate how much total fat, saturated fat, and trans fat a product contains. Saturated and trans fats are implicated in raising blood cholesterol levels and clogging the arteries. You'll find saturated fats in all animal products, as well as in coconut and palm oils. These fats are solid at room temperature (think of butter and shortening). Choose heart-healthier unsaturated fats such as polyunsaturated corn, safflower, sunflower, and soybean oils and monounsaturated olive and canola oil. Here are just a few other ways you can reduce fat in your diet:

• Trim fat from meats and remove skin from poultry before eating.

• Bake, broil, poach, or steam instead of frying. Season foods with herbs and spices, not butter, margarine, or sauce.

• Ask for sauces and dressings to be served "on the side." Then dip your fork lightly in these to get the flavor.

• Make substitutions. Substitute low-fat frozen yogurt for ice cream, skim milk for low-fat or whole milk, fat-free salad dressing for regular dressing.

• Eat more vegetables, less meat. Veggies fill you up and add fiber to your diet.

FIT IN FIBER

By now you've heard all the claims about the benefits of fiber. This is one area where you can believe what you hear. Including a source of fiber at every meal can have the following benefits:

• Fiber helps you to eat less because you feel full faster.

• It adds bulk, preventing constipation and hemorrhoids.

• It triggers less of a rise in blood glucose levels than other nutrients, and the effect remains a while due to slower absorption of food.

• It may reduce the risk of colon and rectal cancers.

• It lowers cholesterol.

Fiber is actually a group of widely different plant carbohydrates that the human digestive tract does not completely digest and absorb as it does other forms of carbohydrate. Fiber is found in unrefined grains such as whole wheat, rye, corn, oats, and brown rice; dried beans and peas; and all fruits and vegetables. Most nutrition experts suggest consuming 20 to 35 grams of fiber each day. Try the following tips for boosting your fiber intake:

• Choose whole-grain breads instead of refined white breads, bran cereal instead of plain cornflakes, brown rice instead of white rice, whole wheat instead of regular pasta.

• Leave the edible skins on fresh fruits and vegetables. These skins are an excellent source of fiber.

• Eat a piece of fresh fruit rather than drinking juice. An orange has more fiber than does orange juice.

• Read labels for the amount of fiber the food contains.

• Drink plenty of water. If fiber does not absorb enough water, it can slow rather than speed up elimination.

KNOW HOW ALCOHOL FITS IN

In most cases, you can fit one or two alcoholic drinks into your meal plan with little effect on blood glucose levels. But do recognize that alcohol's effects may be cause for concern.

Alcohol blocks the liver from releasing glucose during periods of fasting (overnight or between meals), which can lead to hypoglycemia: This effect can last from 8 to 12 hours after drinking, particularly among insulin users. High blood pressure is associated with drinking three or more drinks per day, and people with diabetes already have a high risk of developing high blood pressure. The peripheral nerves (nerves that go to the hands and feet) can be very sensitive to excessive levels of alcohol in the blood. This suggests that nerve damage could progress more quickly with regular alcohol use. Follow this advice if you do drink alcohol:

• Choose "lite" beers or dry white wine. Mix drinks with diet soda, club soda, or water to dilute them. Sweet wines, liqueurs, fruit drinks, or drinks made with regular soda usually raise blood glucose levels.

• Don't drink on an empty stomach; drink with or after a meal.

• Drink slowly. Limit yourself to two drinks.

• Count alcohol calories. Count one ounce of alcohol as two fat exchanges. Check labels for carbohydrate content. If you adjust your insulin to your diet, you probably will need less insulin when you drink alcohol.

• Test your blood glucose before, during, and after drinking alcohol.

18

PLAN FOR PARTIES

Participating in special events with friends and family and taking care of diabetes need not be at odds with each other! But it can seem a bit tricky. If you're going out for brunch, do you call it breakfast or lunch? When should you take insulin? How do you manage a 3 P.M. dinner? Should you eat again at 6 P.M.?

If you control diabetes with diet or pills alone, an occasional deviation from your schedule is generally not critical. If you take insulin, you can plan ahead to fit in the schedule changes. If you are the kind of person who is always ready for a spontaneous party, you should consider a multiple daily injection routine or insulin pump to give your schedule more flexibility.

If you take insulin, and you've kept careful records, you'll be able to tell when your insulin works hardest and when it does not work well. Does the time of the change you wish to make fall within a pattern of high glucose levels? If so, it's OK to delay your meal, or you can subtract one to two servings of your usual carbohydrate servings (fruit, milk, and/or starches) from the meal. Generally, one serving raises blood glucose about 50 points, so subtract accordingly. If you take insulin, another alternative is to take extra insulin before the meal. Again, generally, 1 unit of Regular insulin decreases blood glucose by about 50 points (it also covers about 15 grams of carbohydrate).

If the change falls during a low pattern, you could decrease the amount of Regular insulin you take, using the same rule of thumb described above, or simply plan to eat more. You can also change the timing of the insulin and the amount, but you must plan ahead for it. Contact your diabetes educator to help you work out a plan.

Also consider these tips for planning ahead:

• If you're dining with friends, ask your hosts these questions: What foods will they serve? What time? Will they serve snacks before dinner? If the event is a cocktail party, will food be available? (Consider if any appetizers will be the type you can make a meal out of.) Will they serve dessert at the time of the meal or later in the evening? Decide if the foods available are appropriate for your needs or if you need to supplement them or adjust your insulin. If mealtime is uncertain, you may not want to take insulin until you are sure food is available. Always carry glucose tablets, or ask for crackers, juice, or soda if a meal is delayed.

• Offer to bring a healthy dish or dessert if the planned menu consists of tempting high-fat foods. Put a six-pack of diet drinks in your car in case none is available.

• Follow the same suggestions for restaurant dining. Call ahead to ask what selections are on the menu. If dinner is delayed, ask the waiter for bread or crackers to tide you over. (Test blood glucose if you can: If it is normal or high, you can wait for dinner without a problem.) Again, hold off taking your insulin until the food is served.

• Try to stay within 1 to 1½ hours of your usual schedule. If this is not possible, talk to your doctor about taking intermediate-acting insulin at the usual time and moving the Regular insulin to 30 minutes before you eat. You may need to adjust your dose if you do this.

• Decide in advance how you'll handle special foods and plan for any alcoholic beverages.

19

PAMPER YOUR FEET

Whether you have type I or type II diabetes, it is important to take good care of your feet. The best way to do this is with good glucose control. Like other complications of diabetes, foot problems develop from nerve and blood vessel damage that occurs when blood glucose levels are persistently high for a number of years. The excess glucose coats the nerve cells and narrows the small blood vessels to the feet, accelerating the process that causes atherosclerosis (the buildup of fatty deposits on the inner lining of the blood vessels). Other factors such as a family history of heart disease and unhealthy lifestyle choices (smoking, high-fat diet, lack of exercise) also increase your risk of nerve and blood vessel damage.

High blood glucose levels also increase your risk of infection. Bacteria love to grow on sugar in tissues, and white cells can't battle the infection effectively when they're sticky with sugar. If not treated early, infections or ulcers of the feet can develop into serious conditions.

Nerve damage can develop slowly; you may not even be aware of a problem. Warnings of nerve damage include pain, burning, tingling or a "pins and needles" feeling, or numbness.

Follow these tips to prevent foot problems:

• Examine your feet after a shower or bath. Notify your doctor of any redness, blisters, corns, scrapes, cracks, or swelling. Have the doctor examine your feet at every checkup.

• Wash your feet every day with a mild soap and warm water. Dry them thoroughly, including between the toes.

Easy Ways to Manage Diabetes

- Lower the temperature of your water tank to 120 degrees Fahrenheit. Your bathwater should be about 90 degrees. Test water temperature with your elbow before putting your feet into the bathtub. Your feet may not be as sensitive to temperature, and you could burn yourself.
- Don't soak your feet; this dries out the skin, resulting in cracks that could become infected. Avoid use of strong chemicals such as Epsom salts or iodine in your bathwater.
- Moisturize your feet with lotion. Try products that contain lanolin. Bag balm and udder cream, available at hardware, seed and feed, and many drugstores, are inexpensive medicated lanolin spreads.
- Keep your toenails trimmed.
- Always wear socks or stockings to prevent friction or rubbing of shoes against bare skin. Wear cotton socks; they allow your feet to "breathe," keeping them dry and cool.
- Make sure your shoes are comfortable and the right size. If new shoes are stiff or they rub, have them stretched or softened. Break in new shoes gradually.
- Check your shoes and socks before you put them on to make sure no objects have found their way inside. People with nerve disease can injure their feet because they may not feel objects inside their shoes.
- Protect your feet from the cold. Wear warm socks or fleece-lined boots in cold temperatures. Wear socks at night. But do not use heating pads or hot water bottles to keep your feet warm; they can cause burns.
- Avoid wearing tight socks or garters. Support hosiery is fine because it prevents blood from pooling in the feet and legs. Remove hosiery daily, and wear clean hose each day.
- Wear shoes whenever possible, even at home. Going barefoot increases your risk of foot injury.

20

SEE YOUR EYE DOCTOR

Uncontrolled diabetes can lead to serious eye disease (retinopathy) and loss of vision. It is now well-known, however, that there are two essential things you can do to best safeguard your vision: Control your blood glucose levels and have regularly scheduled eye exams. Sound medical management of your diabetes and regular, yearly eye examinations can all but eliminate retinopathy.

Your risk of retinopathy is related to how long you've had diabetes, your level of glucose control, and whether you have high blood pressure (hypertension). Hypertension increases pressure on blood vessels, while persistent high blood glucose (hyperglycemia) causes narrowing of them.

You may notice that when your blood glucose levels are high, your vision is blurry. This is not a sign of eye disease; it is caused by the lens in your eye changing shape with glucose and water shifts in your body. It usually clears up when blood glucose levels return to normal. People also notice blurred vision for a short time (a few days to a few weeks) after they begin taking insulin. If blurred vision does not clear up, consult an ophthalmologist (eye doctor).

But you can prevent eye problems. Follow this advice:

• See your ophthalmologist at least once a year, particularly if you have had type I diabetes for five or more years.

• If you notice flashing lights, dark spots, or floaters that block your vision, call your eye doctor immediately.

• If you wear contact lenses, be sure to follow your doctor's recommendations for wear, cleansing, and use of saline drops. If your eyes become too dry, your cornea may be more susceptible to injury and, once injured, may not heal well.

ADJUST FOR SICK DAYS

When you cannot eat or exercise as usual, the change in your routine combined with the stress of illness can significantly impact diabetes control.

When you're ill, your body produces stress hormones that cause blood glucose levels to go up and may produce ketones. However, glucose levels may drop if you have nausea, vomiting, diarrhea, or poor appetite. It is crucial to test blood glucose levels and urine for ketones frequently.

Follow this advice during an illness:

• Always take your insulin or medication. You may need to adjust the dose, however. When vomiting is a symptom, you might need extra insulin due to the stress of the illness.

• Test urine for ketones frequently. If the amount of ketones is small, drink fluids and continue to monitor them. If ketones persist or if levels are moderate or high, call your doctor.

• Test your blood glucose every two hours when you exerience vomiting or diarrhea. Test at least four times a day if you have a cold or fever.

• Drink plenty of fluids. Try to take in about 8 ounces of fluid per hour. If you are vomiting, sip flat regular soda. If blood glucose levels are high, drink sugar-free beverages. If glucose levels run low, drink regular soda or fruit juice.

• Eat small meals or snacks frequently. Try foods that contain enough carbohydrate to replace what you normally eat in your meal plan but are more easily digested.

• Consult your doctor before taking over-the-counter cold and flu medications. Some medications can affect glucose levels or produce side effects you may confuse with hypoglycemia.

Easy Ways to Manage Diabetes

Keep good records of your blood and urine tests, food, beverages, and symptoms. Call your doctor or diabetes educator if:

- you have been vomiting or have diarrhea for more than 24 hours
- you cannot eat or drink
- your blood glucose is greater than 240 milligrams/deciliter (mg/dL) or less than 80 mg/dL for more than 48 hours
- you have a temperature of 101 degrees or greater for two or more days
- you have ketones in your urine
- you have signs of ketoacidosis
- you have chest pain
- you don't know how to manage your illness and diabetes

Be prepared to provide the following information:
- how long you have been ill and your symptoms
- blood glucose and urine ketone results for at least the past 24 hours up to the present
- the amount of insulin you've taken
- the last time you ate or drank, what, and how much
- how you have been treating your illness (over-the-counter medications, fluids, and so on)
- the telephone number of your pharmacy

DON'T GIVE YOUR MOUTH THE BRUSH-OFF

High blood glucose levels can make people with diabetes more prone to diseases of the teeth and gums. That's because, most often, disease results from bacterial infection in the gums. Bacteria love dark, moist places such as your mouth, and the higher levels of glucose in your saliva actually nourish them. Infection-fighting white cells sticky with sugar can't fight bacteria effectively. The stress of fighting an infection can cause glucose levels to continue to rise. To sum it up: Dark, moist places + high glucose content = Bacteria that thrive and multiply!

Properly caring for teeth and gums and keeping blood glucose levels in control are the best ways to help your body fight infection and prevent dental disease. Dental infections, or abscesses, are common with more serious dental disease and can cause blood glucose levels to go up. If you have an infection, you may need to adjust your medication.

Some types of dental disease are common in people with diabetes, including gingivitis, a reversible condition affecting the gums. Periodontitis, the more advanced stage of gum disease, follows untreated gingivitis. Periodontitis can erode the bone that supports the teeth.

Here are tips to keep your mouth healthy:

• Brush your teeth at least twice a day. Brushing after every meal or snack is even better, especially if you've eaten a sweet, sticky food. Be sure to brush before bed.

• Floss your teeth every day. Flossing helps prevent plaque from forming between the teeth—where your brush can't reach.

- Use a soft toothbrush and a toothpaste with fluoride. Ask your dentist to recommend an antiseptic mouthwash that can kill the bacteria that cause plaque.
- When you can't brush your teeth, chew sugar-free gum after meals to help dislodge food particles between teeth.
- See your dentist twice a year for cleaning. Make sure he or she knows you have diabetes.
- If you notice swelling, redness, bleeding or sore gums, loose teeth, or a bad taste in your mouth, see your dentist. Call as soon as you feel the first twinges of pain. The right treatment early can prevent more serious problems later.
- See your dentist regularly if you wear dentures. Dentures should be relined from time to time to prevent sore spots and ulcers from developing.
- Give your dentist the name and phone number of your doctor, and ask that the doctor be notified of any problems.
- Ask your dentist to consult your doctor before any dental surgery. You may need to make major adjustments in your medication depending on when the surgery takes place, the seriousness of the surgery, the type of anesthesia, and how well you will be able to eat afterward.
- If you must undergo a major dental procedure, prepare for any inability to chew. You may need to purchase some special foods for your recovery period. Look for easy-to-swallow sources of carbohydrate such as soup, shakes, ice cream, ice milk, sherbet, sorbet, or hot cereals.
- Try to arrange your dental appointments so they don't interfere with your meal schedule. Don't skip a meal or your medication before your appointment.

IDENTIFY YOURSELF

In an emergency it is critical that emergency personnel know you have diabetes. Various forms of medical identification (ID) are available: wallet cards, neck chains, bracelets, or ID tags to place on your watch. Some IDs have an 800 number that anyone can call day or night to obtain computer access to diabetes treatment information. Other IDs simply display the word "Diabetes" or "Diabetic."

• Ask your diabetes educator to provide you with descriptions or show you samples of various types of IDs.

• Choose the ID you're willing to keep on your person at all times. If you decide on a wearable ID, don't buy a silver neck chain if you would be more likely to wear a gold bracelet. Consider any additional cost of a preferable style as an important investment in your health and safety.

• Do not put a neck chain on a young child; the child could choke if the chain catches on something. Plastic tags that pin to a child's undershirt are available, or consider an ankle chain.

• Consider taping a wallet medical ID to the back of your driver's license or identification card.

24

SAFEGUARD YOUR SEX LIFE

Because diabetes is a hormonal disease, it affects the systems important to sexual function: the vascular system (blood vessels), the nervous system, and the psychic (mental) system. Diabetes can alter sexual drive and performance, especially in men. It is well known that diabetes can cause impotence in men, but the effect of diabetes on female sexuality is not well understood. However, some extra care and control can help you preserve your sex life.

For Men

Because diabetes involves the nervous and vascular systems, it can affect a man's ability to achieve or maintain an erection. Psychological factors generally play a role in impotence as well. Use of alcohol or drugs, stress, and depression can also contribute to the problem. If you are experiencing problems with impotence, your doctor may refer you to a specialist for further evaluation. Take the following steps to prevent or treat diabetes-related impotence.

• Improve your blood glucose control.

• Get physically fit. Shed a few pounds. Start a strength-training program. An improved self-image can play an important role in sexual function.

• Seek counseling if you have signs of depression or if you are having problems in your relationship with your sexual partner.

• Don't suffer in silence. Let your doctor know about any concerns you have regarding sexual performance. The problems people with diabetes face are common, and most are treatable.

For Women

Diabetes does not generally affect ovulation or fertility. But poorly controlled diabetes can result in irregular menstrual periods. Many women also report that blood glucose levels run high a few days before the onset of their period. This might be due to hormonal fluctuations or because some women may eat more on those days.

Nerve damage that can result from prolonged periods of uncontrolled diabetes may affect sexual response in women. Hyperglycemia (high blood glucose) may lead to dehydration and decreased vaginal lubrication, which can lead to painful intercourse.

Because bacteria and yeast thrive in an environment high in sugar, women with uncontrolled diabetes are prone to vaginal infections. Yeast infections are very common; symptoms include a white or yellow cottage-cheeselike discharge, itching, burning, and, occasionally, pain. Over-the-counter treatments for yeast infections are available. Check with your doctor before using one of these products for the first time to make sure the condition is a yeast infection. (Your partner may require treatment, too.) If you have an infection, use a condom during intercourse. Otherwise you can continue to pass the infection back and forth to each other.

25

MAINTAIN TIGHT CONTROL FOR PREGNANCY

You're pregnant! Of course, you want to do all you can for your baby. Start by giving your newborn the gift of good health.

It's true that women with diabetes have an increased risk of giving birth to babies with birth defects and illness. This risk seems to be directly related to the degree of blood glucose control, especially during the early months of pregnancy. But with good control of blood glucose levels before and throughout pregnancy, a woman with diabetes can have a healthy pregnancy and a healthy baby.

Maintaining excellent control during your pregnancy can be tricky: Your hormones rage, your weight increases, and your appetite changes. Perhaps more than at any other time, you need to work closely with your health care team to get the support you need to ensure a successful pregnancy.

Before You Become Pregnant

When you are thinking about conceiving, talk with your doctor and diabetes educator about risks to you from pregnancy. If you have long-standing diabetes, you may be at greater risk of developing or worsening certain conditions such as eye disease.

Once you decide to become pregnant, you should determine the roles and degrees of participation of different specialists in your care. Will your doctor oversee your pregnancy and delivery, or will he or she refer you to an obstetrician with experience caring for women with diabetes? You will also need to select a doctor for your baby.

Again, your doctor may wish to refer you to a pediatrician or neonatologist (a doctor who specializes in newborn care) with expertise in treating infants of women with diabetes. Meet these doctors ahead of time to discuss your care and your baby's.

Do your best to care for yourself! Get your blood glucose near normal and maintain the tightest control possible for several months before conceiving. This may require a lot of blood glucose testing, intensive insulin therapy, and strict adherence to a meal plan. But think of what you have to look forward to—a healthy, beautiful baby!

You should also use human insulin during this time. Animal insulin can cause antibodies to form that could harm the fetus. If you use an oral agent (pill), it should be discontinued.

During Pregnancy

Glucose testing, diligent record keeping, and close contact with your health care team are vital. Because most of the changes in metabolism and insulin will occur in the latter half of pregnancy, it's likely you'll need to increase the number of injections you administer as well as the total amount of insulin you take each day. It's not unusual to require three times more insulin during pregnancy to maintain glucose control. Also, because lower levels of blood glucose are normal for women during the latter half of pregnancy, you'll need to alter your target goals. Be sure to talk to your registered dietitian regularly throughout the pregnancy as well. You'll need to change your meal plan as your pregnancy progresses.

LOOK OUT FOR LOWS

One of the problems with the treatment of diabetes with medication—either pills or insulin—is that hypoglycemia (low blood glucose) can occur. Hypoglycemia can occur when too much medication is in the body, you don't eat enough or a meal is delayed, or your muscles use the glucose faster than usual, such as when you exercise. The following are signs and symptoms of hypoglycemia, in the order they might occur:

Mild	**Advanced**
hunger	confusion
trembling/nervousness	combativeness
sweating	disorientation
rapid pulse	unresponsiveness
pallor	seizures
headache	unconsciousness
fatigue or drowsiness	

How you treat hypoglycemia depends on the type of diabetes you have, your size, your symptoms, the actual blood glucose level, and the recommendations of your physician or diabetes educator. There are, however, some general guidelines for treating hypoglycemia.

The first line of treatment is to eat or drink something sweet that will be absorbed into your bloodstream quickly. In a pinch, anything sweet will do, such as raisins, honey, syrup, candy, or icing. However, it is much better to take in a standard amount of glucose rather than devour everything in sight. Anxiously overeating when blood glucose levels are low may drive them too high later. The recommended amount to eat or drink when you experience hypoglycemia is 15 grams of carbohydrate, preferably in the form of 3 glucose tablets, 5 to 6 sugar cubes, or 4 to 6 ounces of fruit juice or regular soda. The amount you need may vary based on your weight and activity level and even from one episode to the next. How quickly the blood glucose level rises depends on the last time you ate, whether you exercised and the intensity of your workout, how hard your medication is working, and whether you ate a liquid or solid food to counteract the low blood glucose (liquids absorb faster than solids).

Plan how you will treat hypoglycemia before it occurs:

• Carry some form of sugar with you at all times. Ask friends and family to carry something sweet, too.

• Don't use chocolate candy to treat low blood glucose. Its high fat content slows the absorption of sugar, so it does not work quickly enough.

• Wait about 15 minutes before consuming more sugar, especially if you have recently eaten a meal or snack.

• Follow the glucose tablets or juice with a combination of protein and carbohydrate, such as crackers with cheese or a small bowl of cereal with milk. The carbohydrate gets the glucose up; the protein maintains the increased level.

• If it's close to meal or snack time, eat your meal or snack. It may help to eat your fruit or dessert first.

• Buy tubes of cake decorator gel or glucose gel (a product designed for people with diabetes). They are easy for someone else to squeeze into your mouth if hypoglycemia makes you confused or combative. Tell family and friends never to force any form of sugar or gel into your mouth if you are unconscious: You could choke or inhale it into your lungs.

- Tell friends or family to ask you a question that requires you to think or problem-solve if they suspect your blood glucose is low. Asking if you are OK is not enough to make an accurate judgment of your condition.

If signs and symptoms are not treated, a severe episode of hypoglycemia can occur. Treatment for severe hypoglycemia is 1 milligram (mg) of Glucagon for adults and 0.5 mg for children younger than six years of age. The Glucagon kit has glucose and water, which is mixed and injected with a syringe. Glucagon is not intended as a self-treatment. It is used to treat someone who is unable to swallow or is unconscious. Store your Glucagon kit in the refrigerator. Be sure family and friends know where it is and how to use it.

WATCH FOR KETONES

Normally, the body uses glucose to feed its cells, which need the sugar for energy to function. When not enough insulin is available to help glucose reach the cells, a process begins whereby stored fat is changed to energy to try to feed the starving cells. One of the by-products of fat breakdown is ketones.

Ketones build up in the blood and spill into the urine. They pull water from the blood into the urine, causing dehydration. They can also lead to a very serious condition called ketoacidosis, which can develop over a period of days or very suddenly with a virus or vomiting illness. Untreated ketoacidosis can progress to a coma. Signs of ketoacidosis are fruity-smelling breath; labored breathing; nausea, vomiting, stomach pain; dry, flushed skin; dehydration (sunken eyes, cracked lips, dry mouth); lethargy, drowsiness.

Ketones develop as a result of insufficient insulin, not from eating too much food or too many sweets.

Pharmacies carry strips to test your urine for ketones. Simply pass a strip through your urine stream, and compare the color of the strip with a color chart on the bottle. If you have ketones, consult your doctor or diabetes educator right away. If you have both ketones in your urine and high blood glucose levels, your doctor may recommend more insulin.

• Test urine for ketones when you are sick. This is particularly important if you have a fever or are vomiting.

• Test for ketones any time you have a single blood glucose result higher than 300 mg/dL or a level that remains higher than 240 mg/dL for more than a day.

• If you have ketones, drink sugar-free soda or powdered drinks in addition to water to replace sodium and potassium.

28

STORE YOUR INSULIN PROPERLY

Insulin is a protein, and proteins are sensitive to extremes in temperature. If insulin freezes or overheats, it breaks down and does not work properly. Follow this advice to ensure that your insulin stays in its proper form.

• Insulin is stable at room temperature for at least one month, so you can carry it in your pocket, purse, or briefcase. Just protect it from intense heat, direct sunlight, and freezing cold; in other words, don't leave it in the car or on a windowsill! Other unsuitable storage spots are the top of the refrigerator and the bathroom medicine cabinet.

• For travel in hot weather, pack insulin in a cooler.

• Store extra insulin in the refrigerator. An area of the refrigerator that does not freeze, such as the butter keeper, is an ideal place to keep it. Store insulin in its box to keep the bottle clean and shield the contents from light.

• Consider warming insulin to room temperature before administering a dose. Doing so may make the injection more comfortable. It also allows the insulin to work within its time frame because it doesn't have to take as long to warm up to body temperature. Although insulin manufacturers recommend that insulin be kept cool, insulin loses only about 1.5 percent of its potency over 30 days at room temperature, an amount not noticeable enough to make a difference in control.

• If you use NPH, Lente, or Ultralente insulin, roll the bottle between your palms or tip it gently from top to bottom to mix it before drawing it into the syringe. The cloudy appearance of these types of insulin identifies them as suspensions, which means their particles may settle during storage and must be mixed with the liquid before each use.

• If you notice a frosting on the sides of the bottles or if the insulin clumps in the bottle, do not use the insulin.

• Do not use insulin after the expiration date printed on the vial label and the carton.

• If a change occurs in your blood glucose control and you can't think of a reason for it, switch to a new bottle of insulin to see if your glucose results improve.

• When you travel by air, bring insulin in carry-on baggage. Don't worry about passing through security as the airport scanning machines will not harm insulin.

• If you need to fill syringes ahead of time, keep them refrigerated and use them within 21 days. Don't forget to roll or tip prefilled syringes that contain longer-acting insulin preparations before injecting the insulin.

• Try an insulin pen. The pen holds a cartridge of 150 units of insulin. You simply dial the proper dose instead of drawing it up in a syringe.

29

BE PREPARED!

Planning ahead will help you avoid unpleasant surprises and stay in control.

• Inventory your supplies at a set time each month, and don't let them get too low. You don't want to run out when pharmacies are closed.

• If you take insulin, keep at least one extra bottle of each kind of insulin on hand. If you break a bottle or something else happens to it, your backup will save you an urgent trip to the pharmacy.

• If you take NPH or Lente insulin only, ask your doctor if it is worthwhile to keep a bottle of Regular (short-acting) insulin on hand for use in special situations when your blood glucose level is high, such as during illness.

• Check your meter case regularly to be sure you have enough strips and lancets. Be sure the meter's code matches the code on the bottle of strips. Keep an extra supply of batteries on hand if your meter is battery-operated. Don't forget to check your second meter, too.

• When you travel, pack twice as many supplies as you think you will use.

• If you are hiking, boating, or are otherwise away from people and food, pack far more food and glucose tablets than you think you will need, especially if you take insulin. Also pack your Glucagon kit and show someone how to use it.

• Always have some readily available form of sugar with you. Keep extra crackers and juice boxes in the car to treat hypoglycemia and a six-pack of diet soda in case it's not available where you're going.

• Always wear a medical ID.

30

LOOK FOR PATTERNS

Learning to identify patterns in your diabetes control is a valuable tool. It takes practice and it takes diligence, but the results are well worth it. Your doctor and diabetes educator will want to see your daily medication, blood glucose, and food records, and they'll help you learn to evaluate them yourself. If you control diabetes by means of diet and exercise, watching for patterns is less critical but still useful. It allows you to see how your blood glucose responds to certain foods and different types of exercise.

To detect patterns of control, you must first have a good understanding of your medication. If you require an oral agent or insulin, know the name of the medication, when it begins to work, when it works the hardest (when the action peaks), and how long it works.

Record periods of activity, exercise, or stress as well as foods and eating patterns. If you had extra food one day or a special treat, write it down. Likewise, it's important to know if you missed a meal, ate lightly, or were sick. Here are some other ideas to help you study your patterns.

• Recognize that two heads are better than one. Study your records with a family member or friend. He or she can help you remember that a particular entry coincides with the night you went to the mall or went bike riding.

• Use color to help you keep track. Purchase two highlighting markers of different colors. Highlight low numbers (less than your target range) in, say, yellow and high numbers (greater than your target range) in pink. After a couple of weeks, study the pattern. When are the highs and lows occurring? Why do you think they occur when they do? If your page looks very "pink" at supper, can you determine why you consistently run over your target range then? Have you been snacking too much in the afternoon? Are certain foods to blame? Are you eating a large midday meal? Or are you eating appropriately, which means you may need an adjustment in your medications or exercise schedule?

- Compare bedtime readings to your dinner menu. Can you track high bedtime readings to certain foods? For example, do you notice that blood glucose levels are particularly high when you eat spaghetti, Mexican food, or mashed potatoes? If you take pills, you might want to experiment by eating less of the foods you suspect cause glucose levels to rise, or exercise longer before or after that meal. If you take insulin, ask your doctor or educator if he or she suggests you take extra insulin on nights you eat these foods.

- Recognize that all foods are not created equal. Some are more refined and as a result are more easily absorbed than others. Some have more fat, resulting in a slower rate of absorption. (The effects of a particular food may even vary greatly from one person to the next.) Figure these facts into your control. If you notice a toasted oats cereal causes a greater rise than cornflakes, choose the toasted oats on an active morning and choose the cornflakes on a less hectic morning.

- Look for a pattern of low blood glucose after exercise. If such a pattern occurs, how long after exercise does it occur? Are blood glucose levels too low in the morning when you exercise the evening before? If so, consider eating a little extra at bedtime, or talk to your educator or doctor about changing your diet, medication dose, or medication timing.

• Look for a pattern of high blood glucose after low results. This effect is commonly called a rebound, or Somogyi, effect; it occurs when hormones kick in to raise blood glucose when it is too low. Because the hormones continue to work for a while after blood glucose returns to normal, a high blood glucose level often follows. On the other hand, high blood glucose levels that occur after low ones may also be due to overeating or anxiety eating. Evaluating patterns helps you identify the difference.

• Keep a record of where you inject insulin. Some people notice differences in their glucose levels when they inject insulin in their arm compared with days they use their leg or abdomen.

• Look for bumps at your injection sites. Called hypertrophies, these raised areas may appear if you give your injections in the same places for a long time. They act like sponges, soaking up the insulin and preventing it from getting into the body at its usual rate.

31

ADVOCATE FOR YOUR NEEDS ON THE JOB

Diabetes is considered a disability under the Americans with Disabilities Act of 1990. It states that "reasonable accommodation" must be made for persons with disabilities. This includes making existing facilities accessible to employees with disabilities; restructuring a job; modifying the work schedule; acquiring new or modifying existing equipment or devices; and modifying examinations, training materials, or policies to make them appropriate for individuals with disabilities. The employer, however, need not provide accommodation if doing so would be significantly difficult or expensive. The Equal Employment Opportunity Commission (EEOC) investigates complaints of violations of the Act.

These tips will help you manage diabetes at work.

• Make sure a supervisor or coworker knows you have diabetes, how you treat it, and where you keep your supplies.

• Tell your employer what you need in order to manage diabetes. If you need to eat a snack or take your lunch at a certain time, for example, let your employer know this.

• If altering a work schedule is problematic, you may be able to change your diabetes management schedule. For example, if you can't take lunch at noon, you may be able to adjust your insulin or add a snack in the morning.

• Keep your diabetes supplies close by. If you need to test during the day, you can do it inconspicuously at your desk.

• If you believe you are being discriminated against because you have diabetes, call the EEOC office at 1-800-669-4000.

32

DRIVE SAFELY

When hypoglycemia occurs, the brain, deprived of glucose, cannot function properly. Clouded judgment, impaired reaction time, confusion, and disorientation can result. Obviously, this is not a good state to be in while driving.

Take precautions before you get behind the wheel:

• Always test your blood glucose level before you drive. Carry testing equipment with you.

• Always carry a form of fast-acting sugar as well as a follow-up snack containing protein. Keep extras handy for times when you're caught in rush hour traffic or the car breaks down. Store peanut butter crackers, juice boxes, and glucose tablets in the glove compartment. And don't forget to replace any food supplies you use.

• If you experience hypoglycemia symptoms, pull off the road and wait until your blood glucose level returns to normal range and your symptoms have ended.

• Drive with a companion when possible.

• If you are the driver on a long trip, you may reduce your calories by 100 the day(s) you are in the car. When you hit big-city traffic, make sure you have an extra snack to prevent low blood glucose that could result from stress.

• Stop to test your blood glucose at 3- to 4-hour intervals or any time you suspect hypoglycemia.

Don't leave insulin unprotected in your vehicle while you're sightseeing or dining, especially on a very hot or cold day. A change in the potency could occur even though the insulin may not look any different. Use a thermos or insulated travel pack to store insulin safely.

33

CARPE DIEM: SEIZE THE DAY!

Don't let diabetes become an excuse. Don't let it keep you from doing what you should and want to do. Yes, taking care of diabetes requires time, energy, and lots of focus. But once you learn to fit diabetes into your lifestyle, it should not get in the way of activities you really want to pursue. In fact, diabetes can give you a heightened appreciation of your health and the strong desire to keep it. It may lead you to see how precious every moment is.

Living with diabetes can also help you keep your priorities straight. We all have responsibilities and commitments. But too many of us spend what little free time we have worrying about problems we can't solve and performing activities we don't find fulfilling. Make time for activities you enjoy! It is not selfish to do what makes you feel happy and fulfilled. Taking care of yourself, preserving your health, and seeking satisfaction in daily life are the best gifts you can give to those you care about and those who care about you. Do what you need and want to do. And take care of diabetes along the way.